Richard Roundtree

RICHARD ROUNDTREE:

The Actor-Unveiling The Modern Impact of The Iconic Legend of Hollywood

Everett M. Goff

TABLE OF CONTENTS

INTRODUCTION

There are people whose presence is both iconic and transformative in the vast fabric of Hollywood history. These are the legends who, with their charisma and talent, leave a legacy that very few others could ever hope to follow. Amidst this remarkable assembly comes a guy whose name embodies all that is cool, a generation-spanning icon of cinematic excellence: Richard Roundtree.

Speaking of Hollywood legends frequently evokes visions of legendary characters who have made a lasting impression on the silver screen. This kind of legend is personified by Richard Roundtree, with his trademark sunglasses and iconic portrayal of John Shaft. But to sum up his life only in terms of his legendary performance as Shaft would be to ignore the extraordinary and simultaneously captivating and inspirational journey of the man behind the shades.

Richard Roundtree was born in New Rochelle, New York, on July 9, 1942, and had a modest upbringing. Growing up in a modest family, he encountered hardships and impediments that would have discouraged many. However, it was precisely these difficulties that helped him develop the fortitude and character strength that would become the cornerstone of his remarkable career.

There was a dramatic change in the film industry in 1971. Following the premiere of "Shaft," Richard Roundtree entered the Hollywood scene in a manner never previously witnessed. Roundtree transformed the blaxploitation genre as the mysterious and dapper private investigator John Shaft, who also became a symbol of black audiences' empowerment.

With his revolutionary performance as Shaft and his enduring contributions to the world of film and television, Richard Roundtree has attained iconic status.

This book, "Richard Roundtree: Hollywood Legend," aims to take you on a trip through his life and career. We will examine Richard Roundtree's personal and professional life, noting the significance of his enduring persona, his impact on black cinema, and his incredible fortitude in the face of hardship.

Through the pages of this book, you will meet the man who brought Shaft to life as well as the performer who went beyond a single part to become an inspiration and a source of strength. The narrative of Richard Roundtree is one of overcoming hardship, shattering stereotypes, and making a lasting impression on the entertainment industry.

Come along on this journey through the life of a Hollywood star who demonstrated that anyone can rise from modest beginnings to become a lasting symbol of cool in the annals of Hollywood history with skill, perseverance, and just the right amount of swagger. The film Richard Roundtree: Hollywood Legend honors an incredible life and career that have enthralled audiences and motivated generations.

CHAPTER 1: WHO IS RICHARD ROUNDTREE

American actor and model Richard Roundtree (1942–2023) is most remembered for playing private investigator John Shaft in the blaxploitation film Shaft (1971) and its four sequels. He was also well-known for his parts in television series like Desperate Housewives, Generations, and Roots and for his performances in other films like Super Fly T.N.T.

For its time, Roundtree's portrayal of Shaft was revolutionary. He was among the first well-known performers in Hollywood to portray a powerful, self-assured, and seductive black character. Many young black Americans looked up to Shaft, and the movie changed the way black men were portrayed in Hollywood productions.

Roundtree was a gifted and captivating actor who will always be associated with his legendary portrayal of John Shaft. In the entertainment sector, he was a trailblazer as well, breaking down boundaries for black performers and directors with his work.

1.1 Early Life

On July 9, 1942, Richard Roundtree was born in New Rochelle, New York. John Roundtree and Kathryn Watkins were his parents. His two younger brothers were Michael and David.

Roundtree started off as a model in New York City. Eunice Johnson of Ebony magazine quickly signed him, and he started to appear in commercials for brands like Salem cigarettes and Duke hair oil from Johnson Products.

Roundtree became a member of the theater group Negro Ensemble Company in 1967, which presented plays written by and about African Americans. In the company's off-Broadway rendition of The Great White Hope, which starred James Earl Jones, he made his stage debut.

Roundtree had a difficult and challenging early career. To support himself, he took on a variety of odd jobs, and he frequently went months without receiving a consistent income. He persisted in being committed to his art, though, and eventually found success with his breakthrough performance in Shaft.

Roundtree's upbringing in a black neighborhood in New Rochelle, New York, had a profound impact on his early years. He had experienced the bigotry and injustice that African Americans endured during the 1950s and 1960s. His acting was influenced by these experiences, which enabled him to play a character like John Shaft—strong, self-assured, and not afraid to defend himself.

As a pioneer in the entertainment business, Roundtree's contributions aided in the removal of obstacles facing black actors and directors. In addition to being a gifted and captivating actor, he will always be known for playing the legendary John Shaft.

1.2 Background

On July 9, 1942, Richard Roundtree was born in New Rochelle, New York. He was the child of nurse Kathryn Watkins and garbage collector John Roundtree. Roundtree's younger brothers were Michael and David.

Roundtree played football for the football squad at New Rochelle High School. After graduating in 1961, he went to Southern Illinois University on an athletic scholarship. But in 1963, he left college to pursue a career in acting and modeling.

Roundtree started off as a model in New York City. Eunice Johnson of Ebony magazine quickly signed him, and he started to appear in commercials for brands like Salem cigarettes and Duke hair oil from Johnson Products. Roundtree became a member of the theater group Negro Ensemble Company in 1967, which presented plays written by and about African Americans. In the company's off-Broadway rendition of The Great White Hope, which starred James Earl Jones, he made his stage debut.

Roundtree's big break came in the 1971 Gordon Parks-directed movie Shaft. In the film, Roundtree portrayed the title character, a private investigator hired to locate the kidnapped daughter of a prominent Harlem criminal. With the critical and financial success of Shaft, Roundtree shot to fame.

In a number of follow-ups, including Shaft's Big Score! (1972), Shaft in Africa (1973), and Shaft (2000), Roundtree played Shaft once more. In addition, he acted in several more popular movies, such as Friday Foster (1975), Hell Up in Harlem (1973), and Super Fly T.N.T. (1973).

Throughout his career, Roundtree remained an actor, making appearances in television series and movies like Desperate Housewives, Generations, and Roots. In addition, he held positions on the boards of directors of numerous large companies and was a strong supporter of equality and social justice.

At the age of 81, Richard Roundtree passed away on October 24, 2023. His contributions to the entertainment industry helped break down barriers for black actors and filmmakers. He was a pioneer in this field. In addition to being a gifted and captivating actor, he will always be known for playing the legendary John Shaft.

1.3 Rising to Fame

Richard Roundtree became well-known in 1971 after landing the lead role in the movie Shaft. With the critical and financial success of the movie, Roundtree shot to fame. There were various reasons why Shaft was a pioneering movie. It was among the first significant Hollywood productions with a black actor playing the lead role and among the first to represent the black experience in America accurately. Because of Roundtree's legendary portrayal of Shaft, the character has come to represent black empowerment and pride.

A number of things played a part in Roundtree's ascent to prominence. He was, first and foremost, a gifted and endearing actor. He exuded confidence and coolness in the part of Shaft and had a natural presence on television. Second, the movie's release window was ideal. Amidst significant social and political shifts in the United States throughout the late 1960s and early 1970s, viewers were keen to watch movies that captured the essence of the shifting society. Thirdly, Shaft has a superb cast and a well-written screenplay, making it a well-made movie.

Roles in other popular movies, including Super Fly T.N.T. (1973), Hell Up in Harlem (1973), and Friday Foster (1975), came Roundtree's way after his breakthrough in Shaft. In addition, he made appearances in several well-known TV series, such as Desperate Housewives, Generations, and Roots.

Roundtree's ascent to prominence was noteworthy for a number of reasons. He was among the first black actors in Hollywood to become widely successful. Second, his accomplishments made it easier for other black actors and filmmakers to enter the business. Third, he changed the perception of black men in popular culture with his legendary performance as Shaft.

Future generations will be inspired and amused by the legacy of Richard Roundtree, a pioneer in the entertainment sector.

CHAPTER 2: THE BIRTH OF AN ICON

Richard Roundtree became a legend after he starred in the 1971 movie Shaft. Gordon Parks and Ernest Tidyman penned the novel for this ground-breaking blaxploitation movie, which told the tale of John Shaft, a private eye hired to free the kidnapped daughter of a prominent Harlem criminal. Roundtree gave a legendary performance as Shaft. He exuded charm, confidence, and coolness, and he gave the part a feeling of authority and dignity.

Shaft established Roundtree as a household name and was a critical and financial triumph. His persona served as an inspiration to a new wave of black performers and filmmakers, and he came to represent black empowerment and pride. In two follow-ups, Shaft's Big Score! (1972) and Shaft in Africa (1973), Roundtree played Shaft again. He also featured in several more hit movies, including Super Fly T.N.T. Because of

Roundtree's performance in Shaft, black men's representation in Hollywood movies was altered. Before Shaft, black men were frequently stereotyped as violent thugs or submissive servants. But Roundtree's Shaft was a multifaceted, clever, smart, and competent guy. He served as an inspiration to black men and women worldwide and contributed to dispelling the long-standing racist myths that Hollywood had been feeding for many years.

The fact that Roundtree's birth coincided with a period of profound social and political upheaval in the US added more significance to his icon status. Black Americans demanded equal rights and treatment under the law during the height of the Civil Rights Movement in the late 1960s and early 1970s. With his portrayal of Shaft,

Roundtree demonstrated that progress was being achieved, and he encouraged many African Americans to follow their aspirations and realize their full potential.

A real legend, Richard Roundtree paved the path for future black performers and directors to succeed in Hollywood through his body of work. He is an inspiration to all of us, and future generations will draw inspiration from his legacy.

2.1 Shaft (1971): An Innovative Role

John Shaft, played by Richard Roundtree in the 1971 movie For a number of reasons, Shaft was a breakthrough performance. First of all, the film was among the first big Hollywood productions to cast a black actor in the title role. Second, Shaft was a brilliant, resourceful, and competent guy who was multifaceted and well-rounded. This was a change from the way black men had previously been portrayed in Hollywood movies, where they were frequently portrayed as deadly thugs or servile servant clichés. Thirdly, the movie's commercial success opened doors for more black performers and directors to follow in Hollywood.

A private investigator hired by a prominent Harlem criminal family to save his daughter, who had been abducted, was Roundtree's Shaft, a calm, self-assured, and charming man. On top of that, he was a man of principles, willing to risk his own life to defend his convictions. Due to his highly regarded performance, Roundtree received a Golden Globe nomination for Best Actor in a Motion Picture Drama.

Shaft was a commercial and critical hit as well. It was the highest-grossing movie of 1971 and inspired a TV show as well as two sequels. Roundtree's career took off as a result of the movie's success, and he went on to feature in several other hit movies, including Friday Foster (1975), Super Fly T.N.T.

One of the most significant moments for black actors in Hollywood was Roundtree's portrayal of Shaft. It changed the way that black men were portrayed in Hollywood movies and demonstrated that black performers could be successful in main roles. Actors and filmmakers are still motivated by Roundtree's legacy from Shaft today.

2.2 Significance to Culture

There is no denying Richard Roundtree's cultural significance. He was among the first black performers to become well-known in Hollywood, and his memorable portrayal of John Shaft altered the perception of black men in popular culture.

A private investigator hired by a prominent Harlem criminal family to save his daughter, who had been abducted, was Roundtree's Shaft, a calm, self-assured, and charming man. On top of that, he was a man of principles, willing to risk his own life to defend his convictions. Due to his highly regarded performance, Roundtree received a Golden Globe nomination for Best Actor in a Motion Picture Drama.

Shaft was a commercial and critical hit as well. It was the highest-grossing movie of 1971 and inspired a TV show as well as two sequels. Roundtree's career took off as a result of the movie's success, and he went on to feature in several other hit movies, including Friday Foster (1975),

The cultural relevance of Roundtree extends beyond his performance career. In addition, he was a prosperous businessman and philanthropist. He was a founding member of the production business Roundtree Entertainment and a director of several large corporations. Additionally, he was a strong supporter of equality and social justice.

2.3 Impact

He contributed to the blaxploitation genre's rise to popularity, which allowed black performers and filmmakers to tell their own stories and depict black characters in a more nuanced and realistic manner.

Actors of African descent such as Denzel Washington, Samuel L. Jackson, and Will Smith were influenced by him.

He contributed to the transformation of black males from docile caricatures into strong, multifaceted characters in Hollywood movies.

He was an outspoken supporter of racial equality and civil rights who used his platform to speak out on social and political concerns.

He served as an inspiration for black men and women worldwide, fostering a sense of black empowerment and pride.

2.4 Remakes

Three follow-ups to the 1971 original Shaft, starring Richard Roundtree: Shaft's Big Score! (1972)

Africa's Shaft (1973)

Shaft in 2000

Two years after the events of the previous movie, Shaft's Big Score! follows Shaft as he looks into the death of a Harlem priest. The movie was a box office and critical hit, solidifying Roundtree's place in Hollywood's elite cast of actors.

Shaft in Africa chronicles Shaft's journey to Africa in order to look into the disappearance of a prosperous businessman. Despite being less popular than its predecessor, the movie is nevertheless regarded as a cult masterpiece.

Samuel L. Jackson plays the title role in the 2000 remake of the original movie Shaft. As Shaft's father, John Shaft

Sr., Roundtree plays the part again. The movie was a box office and critical hit, and it helped bring the Shaft character to the attention of a new generation of viewers.

Roundtree's role in the Shaft sequels is equally as famous as his part in the first movie. In every movie, he has the same cool, collected, charismatic energy. A significant component of Roundtree's legacy, the Shaft sequels contributed to enhancing his stature as a cultural figure.0%Plagiarism

2.5 Offshoots

The 1973 television movie Shaft: The TV Movie is a pilot for a show that was never taken up. The movie tracks Shaft as he investigates a little girl's murder.

A television series called Shaft: The Series (1974–1978) follows Shaft as he investigates murders in Harlem. The three-season show was well-received by critics and viewers alike.

The Shaft spin-offs are significant since they contributed to the universe's and the character's continued development. Additionally, they gave black actors and filmmakers a stage on which to present their own narratives.

There have been several Shaft comic books, novels, and video games in addition to the movies and TV series. One of the most well-known and famous blaxploitation franchises ever is the Shaft series, which has had a big impact on black culture and film.

2.6 The Influence of Richard Roundtree on The Shaft Spin-offs

Both of the Shaft spin-offs were produced with Richard Roundtree at the helm. In addition to consulting on the television series, he produced the television pilot. Additionally, he had a brief cameo in the pilot movie.

Roundtree's contribution to the Shaft spin-offs made it possible for the show's character to stay true to itself. Additionally, he took advantage of his position to advocate for inclusion and diversity in Hollywood.

There is no denying Roundtree's influence on the shaft spin-offs. He contributed to the development of a series and a character that have had a significant influence on black cinema and culture.

CHAPTER 3: THE PERSON HIDDEN IN THE SHADES

The person behind the shades was Richard Roundtree. He was the picture of composure, charm, and self-assurance. He helped to alter the stereotype of black men in popular culture and served as an inspiration to black men and women everywhere.

The 1971 movie Shaft, starring Roundtree as John Shaft, served as a catalyst for the success of other black actors and directors in Hollywood. His legacy will inspire future generations, as he was a pioneer in the entertainment industry.

Roundtree's career extended beyond acting. In addition, he was a prosperous businessman and philanthropist. He was a founding member of the production business Roundtree Entertainment and a director of several large corporations. Additionally, he was a strong supporter of equality and social justice.

Roundtree was a real legend whose life and career served as an example of the strength of willpower, tenacity, and fortitude. He demonstrated to the world that no matter what your circumstances or background, anything is possible.

Richard Roundtree was the man behind the shades for the following reasons:

Cool: It was hard to ignore Roundtree's inherent coolness. Even in the most trying circumstances, he maintained his composure and poise at all times.

Roundtree exuded confidence in both his skills and in himself. Even when others did, he never had self-doubt.

Charm: Roundtree attracted people to him with his captivating demeanor. He was an entertainer by nature and a natural leader.

Intelligence: Roundtree possessed a high degree of intelligence. He had a thorough awareness of the world around him and was well-read and informed.

Compassion: Roundtree was a kind and considerate man. He was a fervent supporter of equality and social justice and was always ready to lend a hand to others.

We are all inspired by the real pioneer,

3.1 Activism

American actor, activist, and role model Richard Roundtree has dedicated his professional life to a number of social justice causes. He actively supported the civil rights movement and took part in demonstrations against discrimination and segregation during his time as a student at Lincoln University in Pennsylvania in the 1960s.

Following his role in the groundbreaking blaxploitation movie "Shaft" in 1970, Roundtree rose to prominence as an African American advocate in Hollywood and utilized his position to support social justice causes. He has made statements opposing racism, poverty, and

African Americans' and other marginalized communities' lack of access to education.

Additionally, Roundtree has contributed to numerous art organizations' fund-raising efforts and has been a steadfast supporter of the arts. He is a member of the United Negro College Fund board of directors, which offers financial aid to African American college students, as well as the board of directors.

Many have been inspired by Roundtree's activism, and he has received multiple awards in recognition of his efforts, including the Black Entertainment Television (BET) Award for Lifetime Achievement in 2009 and the NAACP Image Award for Lifetime Achievement in 2006. He is a real icon, and future generations will be inspired by his legacy.

She began participating in the NAACP in 1965 and has been an outspoken advocate for the group ever since. co-founded the Black Stuntmen's Association in 1973 with the goal of expanding the opportunities available to African Americans in the film industry. established the Richard Roundtree Family Foundation to aid impoverished youth in their pursuit of an education and job training. held a position on the United Negro College Fund board of directors, where they assisted in raising funds for scholarships for students of African descent. voiced opposition to racism and prejudice in Hollywood and society at large. worked to advance intercultural understanding and tolerance. I spoke out in favor of democracy and human rights all over the world.

Roundtree's activism demonstrates his dedication to changing the world for the better. He serves as an inspiration to everyone trying to build a society that is more equal and just.

3.2 Personal Life

Roundtree had five children from his two marriages. In 1963, he wed Mary Jane Grant for the first time. Prior to their 1973 divorce, they were parents to two children together, Kelli and Nicole. In 1980, Roundtree wed Karen M. Ciernia. Before getting divorced in 1998, they had three kids together: Taylor, Morgan, and John James. Roundtree was an extremely private individual who hardly ever discussed his personal life in public. He did, however, speak candidly about his battles with mental health in an interview with Ebony magazine published in 2018. He disclosed that he had sought professional assistance after receiving an earlier diagnosis of anxiety and depression.

Many people looked up to Roundtree as a role model, and he made use of his position to raise awareness of significant social issues. He was a fervent supporter of suicide prevention and mental health awareness. He also made statements opposing racism and prejudice.

Roundtree was a devoted grandfather and dad. In addition, he was a loyal friend and mentor to lots of people.

He was a football player at New Rochelle High School.He was given an athletic scholarship to Southern Illinois University, but he left school early to focus on his acting and modeling careers. His breakthrough performance was in the 1971 film Shaft, but he made his acting debut in the 1968 film The Detective.In addition to a TV show, he starred in three Shaft sequels.

He made appearances in a number of other motion pictures and television series, including Friday Foster (1975), Super Fly T.N.T. (1973), Hell Up in Harlem (1973), Generations (1991–1997), and Desperate Housewives (2007).

He was a prosperous businessman and a generous donor. He was a founding member of the production business Roundtree Entertainment and a director of several large corporations.

He was an outspoken supporter of equality and social justice.

He passed away at the age of 81 on October 24, 2023.

3.3 Breaking Barrier

Beyond simply being an actor, Richard Roundtree was a trailblazer who assisted in removing obstacles for black actors and filmmakers. He was among the first black actors to play lead roles in a major motion picture, Shaft (1971), and his career success paved the path for other black actors to pursue.

Roundtree was a strong supporter of black representation in Hollywood. Speaking out against racism and discrimination in business, he tried to give black actors and filmmakers greater chances. He was one of the founding members of the Black Filmmakers Foundation, a group devoted to supporting black filmmakers and their work.

The work of Roundtree contributed to the transformation of Hollywood. He contributed to making the entertainment industry more welcoming to all people by demonstrating that black actors could be successful in prominent roles.

In order to break down barriers, Richard Roundtree collaborated with other black actors and filmmakers in the following specific ways:

He was a founding member of the Black Filmmakers Foundation, a group devoted to supporting black filmmakers. He acted in black filmmakers' films, including "Hell Up in Harlem" (1973) and "Cool Breeze" (1972).

In order to produce more positive depictions of black people on screen, he collaborated with black actors. He made statements opposing racism and prejudice in the film business.

The work of Roundtree was crucial in assisting in the removal of obstacles facing black actors and filmmakers.

He was a real trailblazer who made Hollywood a more welcoming environment for all.

He was instrumental in the founding of Howard University's Black Film Institute, one of the first institutions to grant a degree in filmmaking. He was one of the original members of the National Black Coalition of Broadcasters, an organization that sought to increase the representation of black people on radio and television. He was a member of the American Film Institute's board of directors, a nonprofit dedicated to advancing the craft and art of filmmaking.

Roundtree's career went beyond the motion picture business. He was a philanthropist and a civil rights activist. He was an advocate for several organizations, such as the United Negro College Fund, the Urban League, and the NAACP.

For all black people worldwide, Roundtree served as a true role model. He demonstrated to them that everything was possible if they put their minds to it. Millions of people found inspiration in him, and future generations will draw inspiration from his legacy.

3.4 Overcoming Obstacles

Richard Roundtree was given a breast cancer diagnosis in 1993. He was one of the most successful black performers in Hollywood at the time, at 52 years old. Both the public and he were shocked by his diagnosis because most people didn't know that men could get breast cancer. When Roundtree was diagnosed, breast cancer was still a taboo topic, particularly for men. He subsequently made the decision to go public in order to bring attention to the illness, having first kept his diagnosis a secret. I didn't want other people to perceive me as weak or less manly." But he came to the realization that, in order to support other men who might be going through something similar, he had a duty to talk about his diagnosis.

Richard Roundtree's breast cancer reappeared in 1996. Although he had received chemotherapy and a mastectomy in 1993, the cancer had progressed to his lymph nodes. Roundtree was determined to fight the illness once more despite being upset by the news. After receiving chemotherapy and a second mastectomy, he experienced another remission. But he lived every day to the utmost, knowing that the cancer may come back at any time. Because of his personal breast cancer experience, Roundtree is a strong supporter of the illness. He urged other ladies to get screened for the condition and advocated for the significance of early identification and treatment. He turned into an inspiration for other cancer sufferers as well. "I'm not afraid to talk about my cancer," Roundtree declared in a 2000 interview with People magazine. It is not a death sentence, and I want people to know that. You can overcome it if you detect it early." Following his second bout with breast cancer, Roundtree kept up his acting and producing career.

He is a real inspiration to everyone battling cancer or other obstacles in life. Richard Roundtree's efforts to raise awareness of breast cancer: In order to support the American Cancer Society's "Real Men Get Screened" campaign, he collaborated with them. He gave speeches to increase awareness of breast cancer at gatherings across the nation. He wrote about his experience in publications and interviews to encourage other women who could be dealing with the same illness. He gave money to fund studies on breast cancer. Richard Roundtree is a genuine advocate for raising awareness of breast cancer. Through his work, the stigma associated with the illness has been lessened, and more people are being screened. He serves as an example for all of us.

Richard Roundtree was diagnosed with pancreatic cancer in 2015 at the age of 74. Pancreatic cancer is one of the most aggressive and challenging tumors to cure. Despite being horrified and heartbroken by the news, Roundtree was committed to fighting the illness. He started receiving treatment right away, which included chemotherapy and surgery. Despite the difficult course of treatment, Roundtree maintained her cheerful attitude. He was aware that he needed to fight for his life in order to protect his loved ones as well as himself. Both Roundtree's surgery and his chemotherapy treatment went well. In 2016, his cancer entered remission, and he hasn't had it since. Due to his personal experience with pancreatic cancer, Roundtree is an outspoken supporter of the illness. He has advocated for others to contribute to pancreatic cancer research and stressed the value of early identification and treatment.

Roundtree's bravery and tenacity in the face of pancreatic cancer have impressed many people.

- **Awareness About Pancreatic Cancer:** He promoted the Pancreatic Cancer Action Network's "Know Your Risk" campaign in conjunction with them.

- He has given speeches to increase awareness of pancreatic cancer at gatherings all throughout the nation. He has told his tale in papers and interviews to encourage others who might be dealing with the same illness.

- Richard Roundtree is a genuine advocate for raising awareness of pancreatic cancer. Through his work, the stigma associated with the illness has been lessened, and more people are being screened. He serves as an example for all of us. Roundtree has persisted in his acting and production career in addition to his campaigning efforts.

Over his life, Richard Roundtree has overcome a number of health obstacles. He disclosed in 2018 that he had received a diagnosis of anxiety and depression earlier in life and that he had sought professional assistance. He also discussed his high blood pressure and his battles with weight.

A few strategies Richard Roundtree used to overcome his health challenges.

He looked for expert assistance. Roundtree had no problem admitting when he needed assistance. He changed his lifestyle to enhance his physical health and sought expert assistance for his anxiety and sadness.

Roundtree was transparent about his health issues. Roundtree was vocal about his health issues in public. He felt that by telling his tale, he might be able to support people going through comparable difficulties.

Roundtree was upbeat and strong; he never gave up on himself. Over the course of his life, he overcame obstacles and maintained his optimism.

The tale of Richard Roundtree serves as motivation for all of us. He demonstrated to us that overcoming health obstacles may lead to a fulfilling life. Yes, that is.

Become knowledgeable about your health issue; the more you understand, the more capable you will be to handle it.

1. Create a network of support. Be in the company of loving and supportive people. They can offer both practical and emotional support while you strive to overcome your health issue.

2. Look after yourself. Aim for a balanced diet, consistent exercise, and adequate sleep. All of them are necessary for general health and wellbeing.

3. **Have Patience:** Resolving a health issue requires patience and work. Treat yourself with kindness, and don't give up if you don't receive results right away.

The life of Richard Roundtree serves as a poignant reminder that one can overcome obstacles related to one's health and lead a fulfilling life. You may reach your health objectives with knowledge, assistance, and self-care He is a true legend whose influence will last for many more years.

CHAPTER 4: EXPANDING HIS HORIZONS

Richard Roundtree was a man whose horizons were constantly being expanded. He didn't like to spend too much time in one spot or doing the same thing. He was constantly searching for fresh chances and challenges.

Roundtree started his own production company, Roundtree Entertainment, as one way to broaden his horizons. This gave him the opportunity to create shows and movies about which he had strong feelings. In addition, he held positions on the boards of directors of numerous large companies, which allowed him to gain knowledge of various fields and viewpoints.

Roundtree traveled the world and broadened his horizons as well. He traveled to numerous nations and experienced a variety of cultures, learning about various lifestyles. He was a genuine global citizen who was receptive to new ideas and adventures.

Roundtree was a more interesting and well-rounded person because of his willingness to broaden his horizons. He had no problem pushing himself and going against his comfort zone. This helped him accomplish great things in life and established him as a role model for others.

The following are some particular instances of how Richard Roundtree broadened his horizons:

founded Roundtree Entertainment, his own production company, in 1990. The company produced television programs and motion pictures with an emphasis on African American experiences and culture.

served on the boards of directors of significant companies: Roundtree held directorships at AT&T, American Express, and Time Warner, among other significant companies. He was able to gain knowledge about various sectors and viewpoints as a result.

Explored the world: Over the course of his life, Roundtree visited numerous nations and cultures. He traveled to South America, Europe, Asia, and Africa. He was a genuine global citizen who was receptive to new ideas and adventures.

Richard Roundtree became a more interesting and well-rounded person as a result of broadening his horizons. He had no problem pushing himself and going against his comfort zone. This helped him accomplish great things in life and established him as a role model for others.

4.1 Past Shaft

Richard Roundtree had a lengthy and prosperous career in addition to his well-known role as John Shaft in the 1971 film Shaft. Along with being a successful businessman and philanthropist, he starred in a number of movies and TV series.

- Super Fly T.N.T. is another role (1973).
- Harlem Hell Up (1973)
- Roots (1977) Friday Foster (1975)
- Generations (1997-present)
- Housewives in Desperation (2007)

In addition, Roundtree starred in a television series and multiple Shaft sequels. He made appearances in several other motion pictures and TV series, such as Law & Order: Special Victims Unit, The Mod Squad, Quincy, M.E., and others.

Roundtree was not only a successful actor but also a prosperous businessman. He was a founding member of the production business Roundtree Entertainment and a director of several large corporations. Additionally, he was a strong supporter of equality and social justice.

Future generations will be inspired by the pioneering work of Richard Roundtree in the entertainment industry.

He demonstrated to the world that no matter what your circumstances or background, anything is possible.

Here are a few instances of Richard Roundtree's influence outside of Shaft:

He paved the path for other African American actors and filmmakers to succeed in Hollywood.

For black men and women worldwide, he served as an inspiration.

He made a statement on significant social issues using his platform.

He was a prosperous businessman and a generous donor.

4.2 Movies

Throughout his career, Richard Roundtree has starred in a number of movies, such as

- Shaft (1971).
- Big Score! by Shaft (1972)
- Africa's Shaft (1973)

- Hell Up in Harlem (1973) and Super Fly T.N.T. (1973)
- Foster Friday, 1975; Diamonds, 1975
- 1973's Charly-One-Eye and 1979's Day of the Assassin
- Vultures' Game (1979)
- Quincy, M.E. (1978–1983) Roots (1977)
- From 1971 to 1973, the Mod Squad
- Law & Order: Generations (1991–1997); Special Victims Unit (1999–2001)
- Becoming Mary Jane (2013–2019) Family Reunion (2019–2023) Desperate Housewives (2007)

In the 2000 film adaptation, he again played John Shaft, and he made an appearance in the 2019 follow-up, Shaft. A true icon of the blaxploitation genre, Richard Roundtree's films have left a lasting impression on popular culture.

4.3 Honors

Richard Roundtree was honored with these accolades:

- MTV's 1994 Lifetime Achievement Award
- 2002 Peabody Award
- The 2010 Black Theater Alliance Lifetime Achievement Award
- For his performance in Shaft (1971), he was also nominated for an Image Award for Outstanding Actor in a Motion Picture.

Roundtree was a trailblazing actor whose blaxploitation character, John Shaft, altered the way black males were portrayed in Hollywood. He was a real icon, and future generations will be motivated by his legacy.

4.4 Recognition

Among the most significant and prominent black performers of all time is Richard Roundtree. His most famous performance was in the critically and commercially successful 1971 movie Shaft, when he played John Shaft. The blaxploitation subgenre was popularized by the movie, and Roundtree's performance was hailed for its swagger, charm, and coolness.

The recognition of Roundtree extends beyond Shaft. His lengthy and fruitful career in theater, television, and film has earned him respect as well. In addition, he starred in several other noteworthy movies, such as Bustin' Loose (1981), Conrack (1974), Shaft in Africa (1973), and Shaft's Big Score (1972). In addition, he had appearances in several well-known TV series, including Desperate Housewives (2004–2009), Hell Town (1985), and Roots (1977).

Roundtree is a successful businessman and philanthropist in addition to his acting career. Richard Roundtree Productions is a film and television production firm that he founded and serves as CEO of. In addition, he founded the Roundtree Foundation, which promotes various charity projects and awards scholarships to students from underrepresented backgrounds.

Roundtree has received multiple accolades and prizes in recognition of his many achievements. He was honored with the MTV Lifetime Achievement Award in 1994. He was honored with a Peabody Award in 2002 for his work on the television series Roots. The Black Theater Alliance Award for Lifetime Achievement was given to him in 2010.

A real trailblazer and inspiration is Richard Roundtree. Generations of black performers and actresses have succeeded in Hollywood thanks to him. He is a living legend, and people will be motivated by his legacy for a very long time.

4.5 Advocacy

Richard Roundtree was a fervent supporter of several issues, such as youth development, education, and stroke awareness.

Roundtree was a fervent advocate for education, seeing it as the essential tool for dismantling obstacles and establishing a more just society. He sought to increase awareness of the difficulties minority students faced and was an outspoken supporter of them. In addition, he gave his time and materials to other educational institutions, such as the National Action Council for Minorities in Engineering and the Roundtree Foundation.

- Youth Advancement: Roundtree was a fervent supporter of youth development as well. He thought it was critical to give young people the tools and chances they require for success. He had affiliations with several youth-serving groups, such as the National Urban League and the Boys & Girls Clubs of America.

- Brake Consciousness: As a representative of the National Stroke Association, Roundtree aimed to increase public knowledge of the illness and its signs. In an effort to assist others, he also related his own experience of having a stroke.

Roundtree's faith in the ability of individuals to effect change served as the inspiration for his advocacy activity. Many people looked up to him, and his contributions have motivated others to get active and improve the world.

The following are some particular instances of Roundtree's advocacy work:

1. He established the Roundtree Foundation in 2003, which supports various humanitarian

projects and awards scholarships to students from underrepresented backgrounds.

2. He was named to the board of directors of the National Stroke Association in 2008.

3. He was selected as a 2010 Boys & Girls Clubs of America National Ambassador.

4. The National Urban League recognized him in 2012 for his contributions to youth development.

Numerous people's lives were significantly impacted by Roundtree's advocacy activities.

4.6 Philanthropy

An ardent philanthropist, Richard Roundtree contributed his time and money to numerous worthy projects. He had a special interest in promoting youth development, education, and stroke awareness.

He established the Roundtree Foundation in 2003, which supports various humanitarian projects and awards scholarships to students from underrepresented backgrounds. The foundation has contributed to the funding of scholarships for students seeking careers in the arts and sciences, as well as historically black institutions and universities. The foundation has also contributed to several other charitable causes, such as initiatives that mentor and support youth and increase public awareness of stroke and its symptoms.

Additionally, Roundtree vigorously backed the National Action Council for Minorities in Engineering (NACME). Scholarships and other forms of assistance are offered by NACME to minority students aspiring to become engineers. Roundtree was a member of the NACME board of directors and a strong supporter of the group's objectives.

Apart from endorsing particular groups, Roundtree also contributed generously to numerous other humanitarian endeavors. He made donations to charities that address a variety of issues, including ending hunger, preventing homelessness, and providing aid in the event of a disaster.

Roundtree's conviction that opportunities and education have the capacity to transform lives inspired his generosity. He was a great champion for social justice.

Here are a few particular instances of Roundtree's charitable giving:

- Since its founding, the Roundtree Foundation has given minority students scholarships totaling more than $1 million. Roundtree made a significant annual donation to the scholarship fund of NACME.

- To assist the youth development initiatives offered by the Boys and Girls Clubs of America, he donated $1 million.

- In order to help the National Stroke Association's initiatives for stroke prevention and awareness, he donated $500,000.

Numerous people's lives were significantly impacted by Roundtree's generosity. His work will continue to help future generations; he was a great humanitarian.

CHAPTER 5: THE RETURN OF SHAFT

The 1971 film Shaft, starring Richard Roundtree, was a critical and commercial hit. Roundtree's portrayal of John Shaft, which helped establish the blaxploitation genre, was commended for its swagger, charm, and coolness.

In several follow-ups, such as Shaft's Big Score! (1972), Shaft in Africa (1973), and The Return of Shaft (1973), Roundtree played Shaft once more.

A follow-up to the first movie, T uphe Return of Shaft, follows Shaft as he looks into the death of a buddy and business partner. Even though the movie did not have the same level of popularity as the first one, it was nonetheless well received for Roundtree's performance.

Roundtree's performance in The Return of Shaft was important because it contributed to the establishment of his reputation as a major Hollywood star. Being one of the few black actors to feature in a big-budget studio picture at the time, he helped break down barriers for other black performers in Hollywood with his performance.

Another reason Roundtree's portrayal of Shaft was significant was that it gave black viewers a positive and inspiring view of black masculinity. Shaft was a tough, self-assured detective who didn't hesitate to speak up for his convictions. Many black men and women looked up to him, and his legacy still serves as an inspiration to others.

5.1 Shaft: Reimagining The Iconic Role

In the 2019 movie Shaft, Richard Roundtree returns to his legendary role as John Shaft Sr. Samuel L. Jackson and Jessie T. Usher also starred in the picture, which was a direct sequel to the same-titled 2000 movie.

Even though Roundtree had a small part in the 2019 movie, it was important because it helped him mentor the next generation of Shaft actors. In the movie, Roundtree's Shaft, a retired private investigator, is summoned back to assist his son, JJ Shaft Jr. (Usher), in looking into his best friend's murder.

Both reviewers and moviegoers commended Roundtree for his performance in the movie. He still had the same coolness and swagger that the character in the first movie did, according to several critics. Speaking about his excitement to play Shaft again, Roundtree expressed his gratitude to be able to introduce the character to a new generation of viewers.

The 2019 movie saw Richard Roundtree reprise his role as John Shaft Sr., which was a suitable way to cap out his career. It gave him the chance to bid farewell to the role that catapulted him to fame and to hand the reins over to a fresh round of Shaft players.

Regarding Roundtree's performance in the 2019 movie, the following critics and fans have said things like this:

"Roundtree is still the man."

"Roundtree is back and better than ever."

"Roundtree is the real deal."

Richard Roundtree's legacy as Shaft is safe. He is one of the most renowned and prominent black actors of all time, and his portrayal of Shaft helped to transform the way that black males were depicted in Hollywood.

5.2 Nostalgia

Richard Roundtree is a nostalgic character for many people. He is well remembered for his famous portrayal of John Shaft in the 1971 Blaxploitation film of the same name. The picture was a critical and economic triumph, and it helped to establish Roundtree's career.

Roundtree's portrayal of Shaft was cool, charismatic, and assured. He was a private investigator who was not afraid to take on bad guys. Shaft was a role model for many black men and women, and he became a cultural icon.

Roundtree's act in Shaft is still highly remembered by many people today. The film is widely acknowledged as one of the best blaxploitation films ever made, and Roundtree's performance is considered to be one of the best of the genre.

Roundtree's nostalgia aspect is also owing to his history in the entertainment sector. He has been acting for nearly 50 years, and he has starred in a number of other important films and television shows. He is a true Hollywood veteran, and his followers respect his passion for his craft.

Roundtree is also a nostalgic figure because he marks a time in American history when black performers were finally being offered big roles in major studio films. The blaxploitation genre was a product of the Civil Rights Movement, and it allowed black actors a platform to express their tales. Roundtree's role in Shaft was a big milestone for black representation in Hollywood.

Roundtree's nostalgia factor is likely to continue for many years to come. He is a cultural icon who has entertained and inspired generations of people.

5.3 Modern Relevance

Richard Roundtree remains relevant today for a number of reasons.

His portrayal of John Shaft is still iconic. Shaft was a groundbreaking character who represented a new and positive image of black masculinity. He was a tough and confident detective who was not afraid to stand up for what he believed in. Roundtree's performance in the original Shaft film is still praised for its coolness, charisma, and swagger.

His work as an advocate for social justice is still inspiring. Roundtree has been a vocal advocate for education, youth development, and stroke awareness. He is a true champion for social justice, and his work continues to make a difference in the lives of many people.

His longevity in the entertainment industry is admirable. Roundtree has been acting for over 50 years, and he has starred in a number of notable films and television shows. He is a true Hollywood veteran, and his followers respect his passion for his craft.

Roundtree's modern relevance is also due to the fact that his work continues to be celebrated and explored by new generations of artists and audiences. The blaxploitation genre has experienced a resurgence in recent years, and

Roundtree's role in Shaft is often cited as a major influence.

In addition, Roundtree's portrayal of Shaft is still relevant today because it speaks to the ongoing struggle for black liberation. Shaft was a symbol of black power and resilience, and his legacy continues to inspire people to fight for justice.

some specific examples of Roundtree's modern relevance:

- In 2019, Roundtree reprised his role as John Shaft Sr. in the film Shaft. The film was a critical and commercial success, and it showed that Roundtree's character is still relevant to audiences today.

- Roundtree has been featured in a number of documentaries and essays about the blaxploitation genre. His work has helped to educate new generations about the importance of this genre and its impact on American culture.

- Roundtree has been praised by artists such as Beyoncé and Kendrick Lamar for his influence on their work. These artists have incorporated elements of blaxploitation culture into their own music and performances.

Richard Roundtree is a true icon, and his work continues to be relevant today.

CHAPTER 6. LEGACY

Richard Roundtree is known for his innovative work, cultural influence, and support of social justice. His most well-known performance was as John Shaft in the 1971 movie of the same name, which revolutionized the way black males were portrayed in Hollywood. The coolness, charm, and swagger of Roundtree's performance won accolades, and Shaft immediately rose to fame as a cultural icon.

Roundtree's performance in Shaft paved the path for other African American actors to play prominent parts in big-budget studio productions. In addition, he was a strong supporter of social justice, and generations of people have been motivated to pursue equality by his efforts. Roundtree is not just an accomplished actor but also a prosperous businessman and philanthropist. Richard Roundtree Productions is a film and television production firm that he founded and serves as CEO of. In addition, he founded the Roundtree Foundation, which promotes various charity projects and awards scholarships to students from underrepresented backgrounds.

Roundtree left behind a legacy of enduring influence. People all across the world are still inspired and entertained by his work, which makes him a true pioneer and role model. The following are some significant ways that Roundtree's legacy has influenced the modern world:

He contributed to redefining how black males were portrayed in the film industry. The portrayal of Roundtree as John Shaft subverted the clichés of black males as criminals or serviles. Shaft, on the other hand, was a black man who was powerful, self-reliant, and assured of his future. Roundtree's performance changed the perception of black men in American culture and paved the path for other black actors to play prominent parts in big-budget studio productions.

He was an outspoken supporter of social justice. Roundtree spoke out against racism and inequality, using his celebrity position. He advocated for social justice throughout his career and was a supporter of the Civil Rights Movement. Through its advocacy activities, Roundtree has inspired others to fight for change and helped bring key concerns to the public's attention.

He was a prosperous businessman and a generous donor. Richard Roundtree Productions is a film and television production firm that Roundtree founded and serves as CEO of. In addition, he founded the Roundtree Foundation, which promotes various charity projects and awards scholarships to students from under represented backgrounds. Roundtree's accomplishments in business and philanthropy are evidence of his diligence and hard work. It serves as motivation for those who are pursuing their own goals.

A real icon and role model is Richard Roundtree. His achievements are groundbreaking; he has influenced culture; and he advocates for social justice. People all throughout the world are still inspired by his work, which has contributed to shaping the world in which we currently live.

6.1 Appearance

American society in general and the entertainment sector in particular have greatly benefited from Richard Roundtree's contributions.

His performance as John Shaft revolutionized the way black men were portrayed in Hollywood. Black men were frequently represented as crooks, sidekicks, or submissive characters before Shaft. Strong, self-reliant, and self-assured, Shaft was a black man in charge of his own fate. Many black men and women looked up to him as a role model, and he was instrumental in changing the perception of black men in American society.

His contributions to the blaxploitation genre increased the chances for black performers to play prominent parts in big-budget studio productions. The Civil Rights Movement gave rise to the blaxploitation genre, which allowed black actors to create their own stories on screen. Other black actors' success in Hollywood was facilitated by Roundtree's efforts in this genre.

Generations have been motivated to fight for social justice by his campaigning activities. Roundtree has made a strong case for youth development, education, and stroke awareness. He has also made statements opposing inequality and racism. Others have been motivated to change the world and become involved in social justice issues through his work.

Other celebrities and artists have also been influenced by Roundtree. For instance, Kendrick Lamar and Beyoncé have both acknowledged that Roundtree influenced their work. Numerous other movies and TV series have made reference to Roundtree's portrayal of Shaft.

The entertainment sector is not the only one where Roundtree has an impact. In addition, he serves as an inspiration to many who strive for social justice. Generations have been motivated by his work to fight for equality and improve the world.

Here are a few particular instances of Roundtree's impact:

According to Samuel L. Jackson, Roundtree served as an inspiration for his portrayal of John Shaft in the 2000 movie.

Beyoncé has acknowledged Roundtree as an inspiration and has included blaxploitation culture themes into her songs and performances.

Roundtree's portrayal of Shaft is mentioned by Kendrick Lamar in his song "Alright."

Several other movies and TV series, such as The Simpsons, Black-ish, and The Good Place, have made references to the character of Shaft.

A real icon and role model is Richard Roundtree. Many people's lives, the entertainment business, and American culture have all been profoundly impacted by his work. People around him are still motivated and inspired by him.

6.2 The Influence On Black Film

The influence of Richard Roundtree on black cinema was significant. His legendary performance as John Shaft in the 1971 motion picture Shaft revolutionized the way black males were portrayed in Hollywood. Black men were frequently represented as crooks, sidekicks, or submissive characters before Shaft. Strong, self-reliant, and self-assured, Shaft was a black man in charge of his own fate. Many black men and women looked up to him as a role model, and he was instrumental in changing the perception of black men in American society.

Additionally, Roundtree's contributions to the blaxploitation genre increased the chances for black performers to play prominent parts in big-budget studio productions. The Civil Rights Movement gave rise to the blaxploitation genre, which allowed black actors to create their own stories on screen. Other black actors' success in Hollywood was facilitated by Roundtree's efforts in this genre.

Numerous other actors and directors have shown their influence on black cinema through their work, as has Roundtree. For instance, Quentin Tarantino has acknowledged that Roundtree had a significant influence on his movies. In addition, Roundtree has received acclaim from Spike Lee, who claimed that he "helped to change the landscape of American cinema.

Today's black performers and filmmakers are still motivated by Roundtree's legacy. Through his portrayal of Shaft, he helped other black people in the entertainment world get access to doors that still serve as potent symbols of black empowerment.

The following are some particular instances of Roundtree's influence on black film:

Roundtree's contribution to the popularization of the blaxploitation genre opened the door for further black-led movies like Super Fly (1972), Coffy (1973), and Foxy Brown (1974).

A new wave of black filmmakers, including John Singleton, Spike Lee, and Quentin Tarantino, were influenced by Roundtree's work.

References to Roundtree's Shaft portrayal may be found in several other Black movies and TV series, including Barbershop (2002), The Nutty Professor II: The Klumps (2000), and Black-ish (2014–2022).

One of the real pioneers of black cinema is Richard Roundtree. Through his efforts, black men's representation in Hollywood was altered, and he served as an inspiration to a number of generations of black actors and filmmakers.

6.3 Paving the Way for Upcoming Generations

For upcoming black performers and filmmakers, Richard Roundtree is a real pathfinder. His legendary performance as John Shaft in the eponymous 1971 movie revolutionized the way black males were portrayed in Hollywood. Black men were frequently represented as crooks, sidekicks, or submissive characters before Shaft. Strong, self-reliant, and self-assured, Shaft was a black man in charge of his own fate. Many black men and women looked up to him as a role model, and he was instrumental in changing the perception of black men in American society.

Additionally, Roundtree's contributions to the blaxploitation genre increased the chances for black performers to play prominent parts in big-budget studio productions. The Civil Rights Movement gave rise to the blaxploitation genre, which allowed black actors to create their own stories on screen. Other black actors' success in Hollywood was facilitated by Roundtree's efforts in this genre.

For centuries, black performers and filmmakers have been inspired by Roundtree's groundbreaking work. People are still motivated to fight for social justice and to improve the world through his work, and his legacy is still felt today.

He was among the first black performers to play a lead role in a big-budget studio picture without needing to take on a supporting role.

His contribution to the blaxploitation genre's popularity allowed black actors to play more prominent roles.

A new wave of black performers and directors, including John Singleton, Spike Lee, and Quentin Tarantino, were influenced by him.

He still speaks out in favor of equality and social justice. A real icon and role model is Richard Roundtree. He continues to inspire people all throughout the world with his groundbreaking work, which has shaped the world we live in today.

6.4   Richard   Roundtree's   Lasting Contribution

Richard Roundtree will always be remembered for his revolutionary accomplishments, cultural influence, and social justice activism. His most well-known performance was as John Shaft in the 1971 movie of the same name, which revolutionized the way black males were portrayed in Hollywood. The coolness, charm, and swagger of Roundtree's performance won accolades, and Shaft immediately rose to fame as a cultural icon.

Roundtree's performance in Shaft paved the path for other African American actors to play prominent parts in big-budget studio productions. In addition, he was a strong supporter of social justice, and generations of people have been motivated to pursue equality by his efforts. Roundtree is not just an accomplished actor but also a prosperous businessman and philanthropist. Richard Roundtree Productions is a film and television production firm that he founded and serves as CEO of. In addition, he founded the Roundtree Foundation, which promotes various charity projects and awards scholarships to students from underrepresented backgrounds.

Roundtree left behind a legacy of enduring influence. People all across the world are still inspired and entertained by his work, which makes him a true pioneer and role model. The following are some significant ways that Roundtree's legacy has influenced the modern world:

He contributed to redefining how black males were portrayed in the film industry. The portrayal of Roundtree as John Shaft subverted the clichés of black males as criminals or serviles. Shaft, on the other hand, was a black man who was powerful, self-reliant, and assured of his future. Roundtree's performance changed the perception of black men in American culture and paved the path for other black actors to play prominent parts in big-budget studio productions.

He was an outspoken supporter of social justice. Roundtree spoke out against racism and inequality, using his celebrity position. He advocated for social justice throughout his career and was a supporter of the Civil Rights Movement. Through its advocacy activities, Roundtree has inspired others to fight for change and helped bring key concerns to the public's attention.

He was a prosperous businessman and a generous donor. Richard Roundtree Productions is a film and television production firm that Roundtree founded and serves as CEO of. In addition, he founded the Roundtree Foundation, which promotes various charity projects and awards scholarships to students from underrepresented backgrounds. Roundtree's accomplishments in business and philanthropy are evidence of his diligence and hard work. It serves as motivation for those who are pursuing their own goals.

A real icon and role model is Richard Roundtree. His achievements are groundbreaking; he has influenced culture; and he advocates for social justice. People all throughout the world are still inspired by his work, which has contributed to shaping the world in which we currently live.

Along with the aforementioned, the following are some particular instances of Roundtree's lasting influence:

For his efforts, he has received multiple honors, such as the Peabody Award, the MTV Lifetime Achievement Award, and the Black Theater Alliance Lifetime Achievement Award.

Television, movies, and music are just a few of the popular cultural outlets that have honored and recognized his work.
He is still in high demand as a speaker and social justice activist.

Many black men and women look up to him because of his success, self-assurance, and strength.
A living legend, Richard Roundtree is a true pioneer. People will be motivated and inspired by his legacy for many decades to come.

CONCLUSION

A living legend, Richard Roundtree is a true pioneer. His legendary performance as John Shaft in the eponymous 1971 movie revolutionized the way black males were portrayed in Hollywood. Black men were frequently represented as crooks, sidekicks, or submissive characters before Shaft. Strong, self-reliant, and self-assured, Shaft was a black man in charge of his own fate. Many black men and women looked up to him as a role model, and he was instrumental in changing the perception of black men in American society.

Additionally, Roundtree's contributions to the blaxploitation genre increased the chances for black performers to play prominent parts in big-budget studio productions. The Civil Rights Movement gave rise to the blaxploitation genre, which allowed black actors to create their own stories on screen. Other black actors' success in Hollywood was facilitated by Roundtree's efforts in this genre.

Apart from his innovative contributions in cinema, Roundtree has enjoyed great success in television and theater. He has acted in several well-known TV series, including Desperate Housewives, Hell Town, and Roots. In addition, he has made appearances in several Broadway shows, such as Fences and The Gin Game.

In addition, Roundtree is a prosperous businessman and philanthropist. Richard Roundtree Productions is a film and television production firm that he founded and serves as CEO of. In addition, he founded the Roundtree Foundation, which promotes various charity projects and awards scholarships to students from underrepresented backgrounds.

A real icon and role model is Richard Roundtree. He continues to inspire people everywhere with his groundbreaking work, which has shaped the world we live in today. He is a true legend whose influence will last for many more generations.

The narrative of Richard Roundtree's life is one of overcoming hardship. He became one of the most successful black actors in Hollywood history by overcoming racism and segregation. Generations of people have been inspired to fight for social justice by his work, and his work has contributed to changing the perception of black men in American culture. Roundtree is a living legend and a true pioneer. Future generations will find inspiration in his legacy.